Pet Food and Nutrition

Pet Food Guide: Optimal Nutrition

Emma Addison

Table of content

9. Trends Shaping Pet Nutrition: Hype vs. Health

Introduction;

After the Industrial Revolution and the growth of the middle class in the 19th century, domesticated dogs and cats started to be kept by families with extra money rather than being used primarily as working animals.

In or around 1860, the businessman James Spratt created the first commercially manufactured pet food in England. Spratt created the first dog biscuit after observing dogs being fed leftover biscuits from a ship. It was made of a mixture of wheat meals, vegetables, beets, and cattle blood. Spratt's business endeavour was a success because it satisfied a fresh market need and sold to English country gentlemen who owned sports dogs.

Chapter 1

The Foundations of Pet Nutrition

Proteins

Proteins, which are made up of amino acids, should be the main component of any pet's diet. Proteins help healthy hair, nails, and immune system function, as well as maintaining muscular mass and providing vital energy. Chicken, steak, fish, and eggs are a few typical sources of protein for dogs. Dogs typically like diets with a lot of protein. Cats are also naturally carnivores because they are descendants of hunters. Protein is necessary for body upkeep, muscle recovery, and cell growth.

All the essential amino acids that pets require are present in animal-based proteins, including:

Arginine

Methionine

Histidine

Phenylalanine

Isoleucine

Leucine Threonine

Tryptophan

Lysine

Taurine Valine

For cats, taurine is crucial. They require it for their ability to see, feel, and procreate. Only proteins derived from animals include taurine. Animal-based proteins are broken down and their nutrients absorbed by a cat's digestive tract.

Energy and Fats

Animal fats or plant seed oils are the sources of dietary fats. They make up the majority of your pet's energy intake. Fats contain more than twice as much energy per gramme than either protein or carbs.

They offer vital fatty acids, which the body of a dog or cat cannot produce on its own. Omega-3 fatty acids, for example, are required to:

healthy skin and fur

certain hormones are produced

ingest vitamins

Body insulation safeguards organs

Carbohydrates

with addition to providing energy, carbohydrates also influence reproduction and aid with intestinal health. Fibre is a kind of carbohydrate that has an impact on the bacteria in the intestine of your pet.

Fibre must be fermentable in order for your pet to receive the most from it.

Wheat, rice, and vegetables are all sources of fermentable fibre.

Young, growing cats and dogs shouldn't eat meals high in fibre. Their diet should have more fat and protein because they have high energy requirements.

Minerals and vitamins

Vitamins and minerals must be consumed by dogs and cats. Your pet will get all they need if you provide them a balanced meal that includes protein, fat, and carbohydrates.

Unless your veterinarian recommends them to address a vitamin deficiency, most people don't need vitamin supplements. In actuality, taking too many vitamins might lead to health issues. For instance, excess vitamin A can cause painful joints and brittle bones. Additionally, too much vitamin D can lead to renal issues and excessively dense bones.

Additionally, cats and dogs receive the following vital minerals from their diets:

Calcium

Phosphorus

Magnesium

Sodium

Potassium

Chlorine

Iron

Copper

Zinc

Manganese

Selenium

Iodine

Healthy bones and teeth require adequate amounts of calcium and phosphorus.

Water

Your pet's body contains between 60% and 70% water. Your pet could become ill or perhaps pass away without enough of it.

Your pet must always have access to fresh, clean water. They get some of the water they require from their diet, but not all of it.

Dogs and cats have various amounts of thirst. When dogs are busy, they become more thirsty, so make sure you have water available for them. Dogs may drink twice as much water on warm or humid days as they would on a cold day.

Further more, The vital component of responsible pet ownership that has a considerable impact on an animal's health, longevity, and general well-being is pet nutrition. To provide our cherished animal friends the best care possible, it is crucial to comprehend the basic concepts of pet nutrition. This chapter explores the fundamental elements of pet nutrition, including the necessary nutrients, dietary needs, and variables that affect the food choices we make for our furry friends.

Intake of necessary nutrients that support diverse biological activities is at the heart of optimal pet nutrition. Proteins, carbs, lipids, vitamins, minerals, and water are among these nutrients. Proteins, which are made up of amino acids, are essential for the generation of enzymes, tissue repair, and general growth. While lipids serve as a form of energy storage and help to maintain healthy skin and fur, carbohydrates are used as a source of energy.

Micronutrients like vitamins and minerals have specialised roles to play in biological functions. For instance, calcium and phosphorus are essential for keeping healthy bones and teeth, while vitamin A and vitamin D support normal vision and calcium absorption, respectively. As appropriate hydration is crucial for digestion, circulation, and temperature control, water is possibly the most important nutrient and is frequently disregarded. Pets have different dietary needs depending on their species, age, size, and degree of exercise. For example, growing puppies and kittens need more protein and calories, while geriatric pets may require diets that maintain joint health. Large breeds have distinct needs than smaller breeds, and energetically demanding pets like working dogs need more of it.

Given the vast array of alternatives, choosing the best pet food can be overwhelming. Commercial pet diets come in a variety of forms, including dry kibble, canned, freeze-dried, and raw, and are designed to fulfil particular nutritional criteria. It's important to carefully examine labels, seeking for an Association of American Feed Control Officials (AAFCO) declaration verifying the food's nutritional suitability. Diets made from scratch have become more popular, but careful planning is necessary to make sure that all the necessary nutrients are present. If going this path, a veterinarian or veterinary nutritionist's advice is advised. Similar to raw diets, which imitate a carnivore's natural diet, unbalanced nutritional profiles and probable bacterial contamination can be harmful to one's health.

Pet owners' food preferences depend on a number of things. Personal beliefs, commercial fads, and cultural standards all come into play. The ideal diet for a pet should, however, be supported by data from scientific studies and specifically designed to meet the requirements of each animal. The optimal diet for a pet's unique needs must be determined after consulting a veterinarian. Specialised diets have arisen in recent years to treat particular health issues. These diets include those for canines with allergies, sensitivities, weight problems, and medical illnesses like diabetes or kidney disease. When taken according to professional advice, prescription foods created with input from veterinarians and nutritionists can considerably enhance a pet's quality of life.

Conclusion

In conclusion, promoting the health and well-being of our animal friends requires a thorough understanding of the principles of pet nutrition. Making educated choices about what we feed our pets requires knowledge of essential nutrients, dietary requirements, and variables influencing dietary choices.

The advice of a veterinarian or veterinary nutritionist is crucial in ensuring that our dogs receive the greatest nutrition for a happy and healthy life, whether we choose commercial pet food, home-cooked meals or specialised diets.

Chapter 2

Understanding Essential Nutrients for Your Pet

Dogs require the proper quantities and ratios of elements from six major food groups, including vitamins and minerals, water, protein, fat, and carbs, to sustain their nutritional health.

Proteins: Building Blocks of Life

The basic building blocks of your pet's body, including cells, tissues, enzymes, hormones, and more, are proteins. They are made up of amino acids, which act as the building blocks for a variety of metabolic processes including muscle growth, immune system activity, and tissue repair. Your pet needs have essential amino acids from their diet because their body is unable to produce them on its own.

Sources of high-quality protein are essential for your pet's general wellness. Animal-based proteins including lean meats, poultry, and fish offer a healthy amino acid profile for dogs and cats. Their protein intake can also be boosted by plant-based proteins such those in grains and legumes.

Carbohydrates: The Energy Suppliers

Carbohydrates are the essential wellspring of energy for your pet's everyday exercises. While flesh eating creatures like felines have restricted sugar needs because of their organic cosmetics, starches assume an additional critical part in the weight control plans of omnivorous creatures like canines. Complex carbs got from entire grains, vegetables, and natural products can give supported energy and help in processing.

Adjusting starch admission is fundamental to forestall unnecessary weight gain and corpulence, a pervasive worry among pets. Moreover, dietary strands, a kind of sugar, add to gastrointestinal wellbeing by advancing normal solid discharges and supporting supplement ingestion.

Fats: Past Energy Stockpiling

Fats frequently get consideration for their energy-thick nature, yet they satisfy a few crucial jobs in your pet's wellbeing. Fats are vital to the construction of cell films and assume an essential part in keeping up with solid skin and a shiny coat. They likewise help in the retention of fat-solvent nutrients — A, D, E, and K —

which add to different physical processes, including vision, bone wellbeing, and resistant help.

Fundamental unsaturated fats, like omega-3 and omega-6, are basic for your pet's prosperity. These unsaturated fats are associated with aggravation guideline, which can affect skin wellbeing, joint capability, and the resistant framework. Wellsprings of fundamental unsaturated fats incorporate fish oil, flaxseed, and certain plant oils.

Nutrients: Micronutrients with Large scale Effect

Nutrients are micronutrients that assume large scale parts in your pet's wellbeing. Every nutrient serves explicit capabilities, adding to a scope of real cycles. Vitamin An is fundamental for vision and skin wellbeing; vitamin D works with calcium ingestion and bone strength; vitamin E goes about as a cancer prevention agent, safeguarding cells from harm; and vitamin K backings blood thickening.

Guaranteeing your pet's eating regimen incorporates various supplement sources is urgent to forestall lacks of nutrient. Business pet food varieties are frequently sustained with nutrients to fulfill dietary guidelines. In any case, talking with a veterinarian to address explicit necessities is suggested, especially on the off chance that you're thinking about home-prepared feasts or concentrated counts calories.

Minerals: The Groundwork of Design and Capability

Minerals are fundamental for the arrangement of bones, teeth, and generally speaking skeletal wellbeing. Calcium and phosphorus, specifically, are basic for keeping up major areas of strength for with and teeth. These minerals are particularly significant during times of development, like pup and kittenhood, however they keep on assuming a part in keeping up with bone wellbeing all through a creature's life.

Aside from underlying scaffolding, minerals are likewise engaged with different physiological capabilities. Sodium, potassium, and chloride are fundamental for nerve capability and keeping up with liquid equilibrium. Iron is pivotal for oxygen transport inside the circulatory system, while zinc upholds invulnerable framework capability and wound recuperating.

Water: The Disregarded Supplement

Water is the most basic supplement for your pet, frequently eclipsed by conversations of proteins, carbs, and fats. Legitimate hydration is fundamental for processing, course, temperature guideline, and the end of byproducts. Water fills in as the mode for various biochemical responses and is fundamental for keeping up with regularphysical processes.

Continuously give your pet admittance to perfect and new water. Lacking water admission can prompt drying out, which can have extreme ramifications for your pet's wellbeing, including disabled organ capability and intensity related issues.

Fitting Nourishment to Your Pet's Requirements

Understanding your pet's particular dietary necessities is crucial. Young doggies and cats have different nourishing necessities contrasted with grown-up or senior pets. Dynamic and working pets could require higher energy admission, while those with ailments could profit from specific eating regimens. Working intimately with a veterinarian or a veterinary nutritionist can assist you with planning an eating routine arrangement that meets your pet's extraordinary requirements.

Taking everything into account, fundamental supplements are the underpinning of your pet's wellbeing and prosperity. Proteins, starches, fats, nutrients, minerals, and water all assume basic parts in keeping up with normalphysical processes and supporting by and large essentialness. Giving a fair and balanced diet that lines up with your pet's particular prerequisites is a center liability regarding pet people who focus on the life span and personal satisfaction of their darling mates.

Chapter 3

Decoding Pet Food Labels: Making Informed Choices

Firstly, we need to understand what does it mean so , The owners of pets should be aware of the critical information on pet food labels. It's important to understand any guidelines for ingredients and nutritional analyses, as well as the way in which the values are presented. The designation of the species and the contact details for the producer or supplier should also be noted. To ensure your pet gets all the nutrients they need, you should also pay attention to calorie content declarations and feeding recommendations. Finally, never alter your pet's nutrition without first consulting a veterinarian.

According to AAFCO, a pet food label must have 9 necessary components: These are;

- The Product Name
- Ingredient List
- Guaranteed Analysis
- Nutritional Adequacy Statement
- Feeding Guidelines
- Species Designation
- Manufacturer or Distributor Information

- Calorie Content Statement
- Net Quantity Statement

The Product Name

This should include information on the food's type and target species, such as "Dog Food" or "Cat Food." The components in the food and how pet food makers must list them are also subject to rules and regulations.

When a product name contains a single component, such as "Beef Dog Food," it suggests that beef accounts for at least 95% of the product's weight (excluding water used in processing). Even if water is taken into account, the product must still contain at least 70% of the stated ingredients. These goods typically serve as toppings or treats because they don't provide a comprehensive and balanced diet.

According to the AAFCO "25 percent" or "dinner" guideline, products with names like "Beef Dinner," "Beef Platter," or "Beef Entree" contain beef that accounts for at least 25% but not more than 95% of the product's total weight (water for processing is excluded from this percentage). The foods can provide balanced nutrition that is both complete and all-encompassing.

According to the "3 percent" or "with" rule, the product with the phrase "With Beef" must include at least 3%

of the listed component, in this case, beef. The ingredients that satisfy the requirements may be listed in the product name at the manufacturer's discretion. They can decide to incorporate any, all, or none of them.

It's essential to remember that these guidelines, which AAFCO created, may not be universally applicable or followed by all pet food producers. When selecting pet foods, always verify with your local laws and regulations and consult a specialist.

Ingredient list

The heaviest ingredient is mentioned first in the ingredient list, which is sorted by weight. Because meat or protein is frequently listed first but contains water in its weight, this sequence can be deceiving. The amount of meat in the final product may be less than it was before cooking.

Please be aware that the list of ingredients in pet food does not indicate how much of each nutrient each component contributes. It's also critical to recognise that the AAFCO's definition of ingredients is different from the terminology frequently used to describe constituents in human meals. As an illustration, the ingredient "chicken" in pet food can include bone in addition to flesh and skin.

Guaranteed Analysis

This section lists the minimum and maximum amounts of water, crude fibre, and crude protein. Due to their vastly differing moisture levels, comparing dry and wet foods can be challenging. The values must be transformed to a dry matter basis in order to make an accurate comparison.

Nutritional Adequacy Statement

It is possible that this is the most significant portion of the label because it indicates whether the item offers complete and balanced nutrients. This claim describes whether the product offers a nutritious, well-balanced diet and how that claim was substantiated. It also describes the species and life stage for which the product is intended.

If the food has been developed to satisfy a nutrient profile or if feeding experiments have been used, this statement will give that information. It is best to conduct feeding trials since they offer concrete proof that the meal satisfies an animal's nutritional requirements.

Feeding Guidelines

These are typically determined by your dog's weight, degree of exercise, and life stage (puppy, adult, senior).

However, keep in mind that these are only suggestions and that everyone has different demands. It's advisable to keep an eye on your dog's weight and talk to your vet about adjusting quantities as necessary.

Species Designation

The item, such as "dog food" or "cat food," must be appropriately developed for the species listed on the label.

Manufacturer or Distributor Information

This information consists of the manufacturer's or distributor's name and location. Consumers can get in touch with the accountable party immediately in the event of any problems. The label must contain this information as required.

Calorie Content Statement

The energy content of the food is disclosed on the label in this part of the information, which is often expressed in kilocalories (kcal) per kilogramme or per can/cup.

Net Quantity Statement

The net weight or volume should be appropriately stated in the appropriate units and placed on the lower third of the principal display screen for product information.

Now we will discuss about that food which may be label with same ingredient but actually there is a big difference in it. Likewise,

Pet Food Label as Meal;

A high-quality, concentrated form of chicken protein is referred to as "chicken meal" in pet food. It is the product that is left over after the water and fat are taken out of the chicken flesh, and it primarily consists of cleaned, ground-up chicken parts including bones, necks, and clean pieces from the carcass.

Chicken by-product;

The term "chicken by-product" refers to chicken body parts that are normally not eaten by humans, such as the neck, beak, feet, intestines, and unhatched eggs, but not the feathers. Even while they might not be enticing, these components can nonetheless provide pets with important amounts of protein, fat, and other nutrients.

The chapter acts as your mentor, imparting wisdom accumulated from experts in veterinary nutrition, food science, and animal welfare. You are armed with the knowledge you need to cast doubt on claims, raise important issues, and make decisions that reflect your commitment to the wellbeing of your pet.

At last, "Decoding Pet Food Labels: Making Informed Choices" is more than just a chapter; it's a life-changing experience. Your position changes from one of a passive consumer to one of an active nutrition advocate for your pet. With knowledge of nutritional percentages, ingredient significance, labelling laws, and ethical issues at your disposal, you'll be prepared to make decisions that appeal to your furry friend's taste buds as well as their overall wellbeing. You are not simply reading labels as you return to the pet food section; you are also interpreting the expressions of care and compassion.

Chapter 4

Exploring Types of Pet Food: From Kibble to Raw

When comparing dog diets, there are several factors to take into account, including cost, practicality, nutrition, and most importantly, your particular dog. Every kind of dog food has its own advantages and benefits, so what may be effective for one dog or household may not be effective for another.

Additionally, because no two dogs are alike, they do not all require the same type of nourishment. Age, breed, activity level, and general health can all have an impact on a dog's dietary requirements. For instance, because a puppy is still growing and developing, it needs more of some nutrients than an adult dog who is fully developed

The following are some of the most important variables you should take into account while choosing the dog food for your pet:

- ✓ Check to determine if it is "Complete & Balanced" according to AAFCO's standard; if not, investigate WHY if you are considering a respectable brand.
- ✓ Make sure the top three ingredients in the food are made from meat by choosing brands that use high-quality ingredients.

- ✓ On the other hand, aim to stay away from foods (such as wheat, corn, or soy) that include a lot of filler materials, synthetics, or additives.
- ✓ Is the food's producer open and honest about how it handles safety? This is crucial because the more food is produced, the greater the likelihood that something will go wrong.
- ✓ The type of food you should love for your dog will depend on its age and stage of life.
- ✓ If you need to feed a dog with certain health concerns, allergies, or sensitivities, see your veterinarian.
- ✓ Talking with other, more seasoned pet owners who have

likely conducted extensive research of their own and are able to provide you with first-hand information on their pets and diet.

Dry Food / Kibble

The most popular kind of dog food is kibble, but that doesn't always mean it's the finest. Dry pet foods can be manufactured from a range of components combined and cooked at high heat, depending on the formula and manufacturer. Pick a kibble recipe that is suitable for your pet because 99% of kibble recipes are created to adhere to an AAFCO statement.

Advantages

- ➢ Convenience: It is simple to serve your dog and simple to store (with reduced spoiling).
- ➢ Options: Kibble recipes offer the most choices among the majority of the other forms of dog food.
- ➢ Although there are many higher-quality, more expensive brands of dry dog food, it is much simpler to discover affordable kibble products.
- ➢ Reduced danger of spoilage: Because it has undergone extensive processing, it is designed to have a longer shelf life.

Disadvantages

- Highly processed: To produce kibble properly, businesses must utilise high temps when manufacturing kibble. High temperatures can have a deleterious effect on the nutritional content of food items.
- Synthetics, additives, and preservatives: Due to the high heat manufacturing method and the long shelf life of kibbles, preservatives and additives are required.
- Lack of transparency: Some kibble businesses can get away with lying about the ingredients in their products.

Situations Where Kibble Is Appropriate;

Puppies if you're a new owner and don't know as much about your new dog's nutritional needs.

when eating kibble, dogs that are generally in good health and don't have any obvious health issues

Parents who want the best for their pet but are on a budget only need to look at higher-quality dry food options.

Raw / Frozen

The most controversial kind of pet food on the market is certainly raw. While some people are concerned about how dangerous it is for both humans and animals, its supporters are passionate in their praise of how great it is.

Both the American Veterinary Medical Association (AVMA) and the American Animal Hospital Association (AAHA) officially advise against giving dogs meals based on raw meat to dogs.

Research on this kind of pet food will continue, and there will be spirited discussions as the "raw revolution" gains momentum. Just be aware that some dogs' health can be much improved by eating raw meat, but every dog is different.

Advantages

- ➢ Natural ingredients: Whole, natural foods are frequently used as ingredients in high-quality raw food brands. The majority of businesses state that their raw diets contain no synthetic substances or harmful additives.
- ➢ Less processed: There is no cooking involved with raw foods. If the diet is properly planned, raw food offers some of the finest nutritional value for dogs because it does not need to be processed

in high heat environments and is less processed.

> Most dogs enjoy the flavour of raw food, especially when it contains meat.

> Helpful in treating some health disorders: Many owners say that after switching to raw food, their chronic health conditions have improved. For example, many dogs who consume a raw diet have softer fur, healthier skin, fresher breath, cleaner teeth, and smaller faeces.

> Higher moisture content: Unfortunately, chronic dehydration in dogs (and cats) is fairly prevalent since their diets don't include enough fluids. A food high in water content is

beneficial to prevent or slow the progression of the disease in cats, who are particularly prone to renal ailments. Your pet is getting the moisture they need in part from their meal because raw food hasn't been altered.

Disadvantages

> The main defence against giving raw food is that it is more challenging to handle securely. The risk of infections is always higher when handling raw meats, and it is more difficult to prevent risks with raw food than, say, kibble. You can feed raw food safely, though,

if you take a few easy precautions, like storing it properly, washing your hands, and always washing bowls. Additionally, refrain from kissing your dog close to or on his mouth, and don't let him lick your face. Unfortunately, a dog eating a raw diet can spread bacteria that can kill humans.

> Storage is challenging: Raw dog food must be kept in the refrigerator or freezer, as opposed to kibble or canned food. It's crucial that pet parents plan ahead because many like to buy in bulk or make their homemade raw food in bulk. Sometimes

individuals purchase a completely separate freezer for their beloved dog.

➤ It can be more messy than kibble, and it can be challenging to properly prepare a healthy, balanced raw food for your dog. It is less likely that your dog is missing any necessary nutrients if you give commercial foods. The fact that humans are less knowledgeable about how to offer all of the essential nutritional components in the proper quantities is one of the main reasons veterinarians continue to oppose raw diets, though.

➢ Greater pricing range Feeding a nutritious raw diet to an average-sized dog can cost up to $2.50 to $5 per day, making it one of the priciest options for dog owners.

Situation Raw Pet Food is Suitable For

➢ Giving typical dogs the best possible health
➢ Can benefit animals with particular chronic health conditions, potential food allergies, or sensitivities. If your dog has persistent

concerns, consult a veterinarian or nutritionist for advice.

➢ Owners who desire greater control over the products their dogs consume and a more natural diet.

<u>Cooked</u>

Cooked pet meals, sometimes known as fresh pet food, are a growing trend. More owners are looking for a healthy and secure substitute as they become more concerned about giving their pets overly processed kibble. People are choosing cooked pet meals as their preferred choice because there is still a lot of opposition to feeding pets raw food.

Advantages

- ➢ Natural ingredients: Fresh pet food includes natural, whole food ingredients in its formulas, much like raw food does. Fresh pet food rarely contains extra fillers or artificial additives.
- ➢ Fewer safety worries: When dealing with fresh pet food, many of the safety worries associated with raw pet food are eliminated because all of the ingredients are cooked.
- ➢ Lower heat: Fresh pet food, whether it is made at home or by a company, is frequently cooked

at a lower heat, especially when compared to kibble. This indicates that prepared pet food retains certain nutrients because it is not processed at high temperatures, in addition to maybe being safer because the meat ingredients are no longer raw.

➤ Similar health advantages to feeding raw: Many pet owners who feed prepared pet food notice similar benefits in their animals as they would if they fed raw, including improved skin and hair, less allergy symptoms, smaller faeces, and better-smelling breath.

Disadvantages

- Very expensive: Equal to, if not more costly than raw because it is a more recent product on the market and requires more manpower to produce a finished good.
- Some nutrients are lost: Any cooking of the components will reduce the nutritional value of the meal slightly compared to feeding your pet raw food.
- Storage can be challenging because both prepared and raw pet food must be kept in the refrigerator and freezer. It might be a hassle for many pet owners because of the storage space needed.

Situation Cooked Pet Food is Suitable For

> Pets whose stomachs can be more delicate and who can't take kibble or raw pet food.

> Pet owners that like to have more control over their pets' diets, ensuring that it is natural and minimally processed.

> A potential remedy for finicky eaters, as some food become more appetising after being cooked.

> topping kibble or raw pet meals in a bowl.

Chapter 5

Catering to Special Dietary Needs: Allergies to Ailments

It can be challenging to feed a dog with a particular diet. You quickly learn how challenging it is to locate a dog meal that both meets your mutt's wants and gives him the proper nutritional content when you venture into the world of specialised dog foods.

First things first: it's essential that you understand the particular diet that your dog requires. Currently, I like to divide special dog foods into two main categories:

1. Veterinary formulas : These are necessary for dogs suffering from a particular illness or medical condition.

2. Cautionary formulas : These are not required to maintain your dog's health. However, some dog owners prefer to get them just to be safe.

A dog diet for kidney problems could serve as an illustration of a veterinarian formula. A dog with weak or failing kidneys absolutely needs to eat this kind of specialised food to be healthy.

On the other hand, there are formulations that should be avoided, such those that are grain-free. Even though dogs can eat grains unless they have an allergy to them, some dog owners choose to be safe and exclusively purchase grain-free dog food.

Types of Special Diets for Dogs

Here is our list of the different kinds of special diets for dogs so that you may choose the right one for your pooch.

Low Fat

For dogs who are overweight, low-fat dog meals tend to be used. A low-fat diet is also necessary for some illnesses, such as pancreatitis and inflammatory bowel disease.

Kidney Problems

Regular dog diets are difficult for dogs with kidney problems to digest. You should definitely visit the veterinarian for this one if that is your dog.

You should follow the advice your veterinarian gives you and feed your dog the specific diet they recommend.

Less protein and more water are typically found in these speciality foods.

Grain and Gluten-Free Dog Diets

Over time, the public's view of what to feed dogs has changed. Grain-free and gluten-free diets have gained a lot of popularity in recent years. Grain- and gluten-free diet advocates assert that dogs don't naturally digest grain. So they shouldn't eat grains or gluten, a protein that is present in many cereals.

Modern dogs often have no issues breaking down gluten or wheat. Only if your dog is allergic to certain elements should you take into account such a diet.

Special Food For Dogs with Diabetes

Diabetic dogs are unable to control their blood sugar levels. This is as a result of their inability to manufacture insulin, a hormone that the body uses to metabolise glucose. As a result, these dogs' blood sugar levels will rise.

For diabetic dogs, low glycemic diets are used. These particular dog diets have higher fats and fewer carbohydrates (20–25% dry matter). If your dog has diabetes, it is recommended to ask your veterinarian for a dog food advice.

Sensitive Stomach

In most cases, dogs don't have sensitive stomachs. Only if your dog is sensitive to or allergic to a food component in its diet might he be experiencing runny poops. This could refer to a particular grain or kind of protein.

The best course of action for you is to take your dog to the veterinarian for a checkup so that he can identify which foodstuffs you should not be feeding your dog.

Skin Sensitivities

Does your dog lick, scratch, or bite his skin excessively? If so, he may have skin allergies that need for a particular dog diet. Dog food for sensitive skin has a small number of components. The most typical dietary allergies for mutts are also avoided by the manufacturers of these diets.

Moreover, You must watch your dog to see how he responds to his new diet.

you should pay attention to the regularity and consistency of his stools as well as the amount of food he is actually consuming.

Dogs' special diets might be challenging to manage. But if you choose wisely, the process may go a little more smoothly for both you and your dog. Before choosing a diet, be sure to consult the vet for your pet and give him the time he needs to adjust.

Pet Allergies

Pet allergens are specific proteins on your pet that triggered an allergic immune system overreaction. These allergies can be found in animal saliva, urine, fur, and skin. Pet dander, which are small scales from your pets' skin, hair, or feathers, also contains it.

These proteins are often not harmful. Your allergic immune system, however, perceives them as dangerous "invaders," similar to bacteria or viruses.

Although cats and dogs are the most common sources of pet allergies, any animal may produce them.

Other animals that can trigger allergies are:

Rabbits.

Rodents (including guinea pigs, hamsters, mice, rats, and gerbils).

Birds.

Horses.

Symptoms of Pet Allergies;

Now we will discuss some symptoms of pet allergies. It's important to keep in mind that these signs may vary based on the type of allergy, the sensitivity of the particular pet, and the allergen involved. It's advised to see a veterinarian for accurate diagnosis and treatment if you feel your pet has allergies. These symptoms are;

1. Chronic Ear Infection
2. Gastrointestinal Issues
3. Sneezing and Runny Nose
4. Hair Loss
5. Excessive Scratching
6. Red or Irritated Skin
7. Behavioural Changes
8. Coughing and Wheezing
9. Swollen Paws or Face
10. Excessive Licking or Grooming

Protections

To maintain their comfort and wellbeing, it is important to take preventive measures while protecting pets from allergies. Maintaining a clean living environment comes first and foremost. Dust, pollen, and pet dander allergens can be reduced by routinely vacuuming and cleaning surfaces. Airborne allergens can be reduced by using air purifiers with HEPA filters.

A crucial aspect of allergy avoidance is grooming. Regular brushing can assist in preventing excessive shedding and the transmission of dander, while bathing pets in hypoallergenic shampoos can help remove allergens from their skin and fur. Additionally, preventing the development of allergens involves washing pet bedding frequently in hot water and keeping it clean.

Affect of Pet Allergies;

Anybody can develop a pet allergy.

If either of your parents is allergic to animals, you are more likely to be as well.

Pet allergies are quite common. In the United States, up to 30% of people have allergies to cats and dogs. A cat is more likely to cause an allergic reaction in you than a dog.

Can Allergies to Pets go away ?

Animal allergies may outgrow them, but this is less likely. Even those allergies have a chance of fading and later returning. Having pets won't make it easier to get used to allergies either. Some people may experience severe allergy symptoms during certain seasons, notably during the summer when animals shed more.

Chapter 6

Portion Control and Feeding Guidelines for a Healthy Pet

Portion control and regulation;

We Americans desperately lack portion control and regulation, and not only do our children suffer as a result, but also our pets. Humans may find it challenging to resist the constant assault of advertisements and Happy Meal temptations, but when it comes to feeding our dogs, we have a clear and straightforward responsibility to uphold. Since we are the only ones who can feed them, we must ignore the little voice that tells us that food equals love and focus on giving our dogs the proper amount of food.

Measuring Dog Food

Once you've determined where your pet fits on the chart, decide if weight loss and by how much, weight increase, or maintenance are the desired outcomes. A 10% change in body mass is represented by each point on the graph.

Start by using a measuring cup—the same cup you would use to measure flour for baking—to begin. Not an espresso cup or a Big Gulp cup. 8

ounces of liquid or dry material can be stored in a cup or container.

A cup of lettuce won't weigh the same as a cup of brown sugar since grammes are a measure of weight; the same is true for the various pet meals available on the market.

The amount of calories in each cup of food varies, which is important to know when figuring out how much to give your pet.

So, read the label on your dog food. Kcal/cup of food should be prominently marked, or at the very least, there should be a visible 800 number to call to obtain that information. What are you feeding if it isn't?

To your family, talk. When it comes to portion control and getting your dog to the right weight, everyone must be on board.

You can decide with your veterinarian how much food to feed your dog or how many calories your pet needs in a day based on current body condition, the caloric content in the food you are feeding (and treats, which do count as additional calories and should make up no more than 10% of the overall caloric intake, so factor them in), life stage, activity level, and goal. As puppies mature, their calorie requirements and the amount they are fed will change.

Make the calculations

Next, a little maths is required. Calculate how many cups your pet needs to be given each day based on their daily calorie requirements. For instance, the diet you serve has 300 kcal per cup. Every day, your pet needs 600 kcals. 600 kcal/300 kcal/cup equals 2 cups of food for your pet per day. Put the dog's daily food and treats into a bag using a measuring cup.

For the following 24 hours, feed from this bag. You can split the contents of the bag into meals that will be filling but not decadent. Most animals thrive when fed smaller portions in 2-3 servings each day. Puppies and small breeds may require more frequent feedings to keep blood sugar levels stable. Some dogs can be allowed to eat at will as long as they take frequent breaks and don't binge.

I've utilised a few techniques to assist extend my dog's eating period, turn it into an educational activity, and let them feel full. The Omega Paw Tricky Treat Ball, the Kong Wobbler Dog Toy, and other treat distributing puzzles may delight children for hours while also stimulating their minds and helping to dispense the right amount of dog food.

Recall that exercise also aids in maintaining a healthy weight! Enjoy the last autumnal weeks.

GUIDELINES

Factors that have impact

Both the amount and type of food your dog needs might vary depending on a number of factors.

- Age
- Weight
- Activity Levels

Age

Your dog's nutritional requirements fluctuate as he develops. Your dog requires puppy food for growth and development if he is still a puppy. Senior formulae that keep older dogs active and mentally bright may be beneficial to seniors. Consult your veterinarian about your dog's lifestyle and life stage to determine the best type of food for him.

Weight

Maintaining your dog in top physical condition is essential for their overall health. According to Dr. Callie Harris, DVM, if your dog is not in his ideal body condition, you may need to change what and how much you are feeding him. To assist your dog in achieving and maintaining his ideal physical condition, think about a weight management supplement. In order to rule out any health risks, we also advise consulting with your veterinarian.

Activity Levels

The feeding guidelines on dog food packages are based on typical adult dogs with typical levels of exercise. If you take your dog on frequent runs or hikes, he may require extra calories to meet his daily energy requirements.

However, You can figure out how much food to feed your dog once you've found a full and balanced food that suits his particular needs. You can get direction from the dog feeding chart on the back of his dog food packaging.

Most dogs ought to have regular mealtimes for a variety of reasons. By being consistent with mealtimes, what you give him, and how much you give him, you may aid him in maintaining good gut health and a healthy weight. Additionally, regular mealtimes might help avoid domestic mishaps.

For the vast majority of dogs, two meals per day—one in the morning and one in the evening—should be provided.

Depending on the formula and calorie content, dog feeding levels vary from product to product. Check the feeding guide on the back of the bag of dog food. Regarding unique nutritional requirements, speak with your veterinarian since individual requirements can differ.

Importance of Specific Amount of Food

Providing your dog with the appropriate nutrition can keep him healthy. Overfeeding your dog can result in weight gain, which can aggravate existing health conditions including joint pain.

He will be able to maintain his desired weight and be active if his portion sizes are constant and suitable for his age, weight, and activity levels. Use our physical Condition System to learn how your dog's physical condition is determined by your veterinarian.

Chapter 7

Balancing Act: Homemade Diets and Nutritional Supplements

It may be more appealing to feed your dog a meal that resembles what you eat for dinner rather than giving it commercial dog food. However, it's crucial to keep in mind that a dog's nutritional requirements differ from your own if you want to ensure its good health. Therefore, you cannot just feed your dog a meal that is regarded as nutritious for humans to eat.

Making the choice to prepare homemade dog food requires cautious thought, as well as discussion with your veterinarian about your dog's present health and long-term wellness objectives.

A veterinary nutritionist can also give you one or more balanced home-cooked dog food recipes. When done properly, cooking for your dog may be a wonderful opportunity for bonding and can give them with a delicious, healthy homemade meal.

Before moving your dog from commercial dog foods to homemade food, there are a few things you should know.

Even if there isn't any clear scientific proof to back up the claim that a homemade diet is healthful for your dog than commercial dog foods, there are measurable advantages that make the choice of making food at home tempting.

Here are a few advantages of eating home-cooked meals:

- Whole Food
- Minimally Processed Food
- Variety of Fresh Ingredients

- Individually Tailored Recipes

Whole Food

You can choose whole-food ingredients for homemade dog food that you would eat yourself. Additionally, you have control over where those ingredients come from, reducing your concern for food recalls and preparation methods.

Minimally Processed Food

In order to suit your food preparation tastes or your dog's particular palette, ingredients can be provided in a variety of ways, including raw, steamed, roasted, grilled, and so on.

The techniques you perform in the kitchen will be significantly less disruptive than those required to turn ingredients into dry kibble or canned dog food.

Variety of Fresh Ingredients

You can include a range of items in your dog's daily diet to add diversity and interest to mealtimes rather than providing the same highly processed food on a consistent basis.

Individually Tailored Recipes

Making your own dog food has several advantages over buying commercial food, not the least of which is that it can be customised to offer the right amount of calories and nutrients for your dog's age, weight, and medical conditions.

To fulfil the unique requirements of the dog you love, such as weight control, dietary sensitivities, or sensitive palates, you can choose a combination of fresh food ingredients.

Making a homemade diet for your dog may sound simple, but making homemade dog food is a little more difficult than just giving them protein and vegetables.

<u>Important Things to Remember</u>

Be sure that you carefully assess the following factors to make the best decision for you and your pet:

- A Nutritionally Balanced Diet Must Be Offered
- Find a Trustworthy and Verified Recipe Source
- The Recipes Must Be Followed Exactly
- Use only high-quality, secure ingredients
- The Time Commitment Required to Make Homemade Dog Food
- You'll need to balance meals by giving your dog supplements
- You must gradually switch your dog to a homemade diet.

A Nutritionally Balanced Diet Must Be Offered

Given that dogs' dietary requirements differ from those of humans, it's critical to feed your dog a balanced diet that contains all the essential vitamins and minerals.

These nutrients include protein, fat, vitamins, minerals, calories to support weight maintenance or promote weight increase or decrease. Diseases, malnutrition, obesity, and even death can result from getting too little or too much of any one nutrient.

Find a Trustworthy and Verified Recipe Source

Again, it's critical for the health of your dog to give the right nutrients in the right proportions to prevent excess or deficiency. As a result, not all recipes for general homemade dog food have been examined to ensure that they are nutritionally balanced, even though you can find them online, in books, or in magazines.

To ensure that the recipe or recipes you use are balanced to satisfy your dog's nutritional needs, speak with a veterinarian or veterinary nutritionist.

The Recipes Must Be Followed Exactly

Once you've developed a nutritionally sound meal for your dog, you need to follow to every detail of it, from the sorts of products used to their measurement to the cooking techniques.

Methods of preparation are important because they can alter a food's nutrient makeup, which helps maintain a balanced diet. Examples of this include steaming, roasting, and boiling.

The diet becomes unbalanced when components are added or substituted, such as when chicken is added on top of something else or when beef is replaced with chicken in a recipe, and there is a chance that one or more nutrients may be provided in excess or insufficiently.

You can offer a larger variety of ingredients and still ensure that you are meeting your dog's unique nutritional needs by creating various balanced recipes utilising a dependable expert source.

Use only high-quality, secure ingredients

Many foods are poisonous or unhealthy for your dog, including chocolate, grapes, raisins, and macadamia nuts, to mention a few.

You should be aware of and stay away from certain items when cooking.

You also need to buy ingredients of the same quality that you would. You should be familiar with the source as well. For instance, purchasing ingredients online may result in them coming from different producers or places, which could impact the final product's quality. Keep the source of the components for your dog's food consistent as much as you can.

The Time Commitment Required to Make Homemade Dog Food

It might be difficult to find the time to prepare a healthy dinner for yourself and your family, let alone prepare meals from scratch for your dog.

Meals can be prepared in advance for the week to save time. For example, creating a large batch on Sunday and dividing it into portions for each day's meals would save time each day.

Additionally, recipes can be adapted to freeze well so that large quantities can be prepared in advance and stored for later use.

You'll need to balance meals by giving your dog supplements

Homemade dog food supplements are frequently needed to ensure that the meals are balanced, especially in terms of vitamins and minerals.

Follow any veterinary recommendations to make sure you're delivering the proper amounts of nutrients and that the food is balanced, taking into account any underlying health conditions. Your doctor can also recommend various brands and offer advice on the kind of dog vitamins you should take.

You must gradually switch your dog to a homemade diet

When converting from commercial food to a homemade diet or even when adjusting the components in a homemade diet, some dogs may experience intestinal pain.

Change your dog's diet gradually over a minimum of a few days to give his stomach time to become used to the new food.

If your pet exhibits any symptoms of decreased appetite, nausea, vomiting, or a change in faeces, call your veterinarian right once.

Chapter 8

Ensuring Pet Food Safety: From Production to Bowl

It's common to think about human-consumed foods when discussing food safety, but pet food processing safety is also important because animals can become sick or even die from contaminated food.

Pet food can be exposed to several kinds of bacteria and other types of contamination without proper food safety and sanitation precautions, rendering it unsuitable for human consumption. Particularly when it comes to the manufacturing of food, animals should be subject to the same safety considerations as humans.

Importance of Safety of Pet Food

Food recalls in the food and beverage manufacturing sector have increased as detection technology has improved. The bulk of them are caused by bacterial contamination, which occurs in both human and pet food processing plants.

The main bacteria behind recalls are Salmonella, Listeria, and E. Coli, and depending on the type and level of contamination, each one can result in varied degrees of disease. Contamination can lead pets to fall seriously ill or even pass away if basic sanitation procedures are not followed.

This is expensive for facilities as well as owners who must pay veterinary fees. Recalls can result in facility losses as well as other negative effects, such as a decline in customer confidence.

Methods to Enhance Pet Food Sanitization

Now we will discuss some methods which enhance pet food safety. These are;

- Schedule Time for Employee Training
- Store Ingredients Properly
- Set up Appropriate Floor Drainage
- Ensure that the space is Clean
- Apply Best Practices For Layout

Schedule Time for Employee Training

In order to ensure that workers understand the manufacturing process and how to maintain a hygienic environment in order to stop the spread of bacteria and pollution, proper training is important. Facilities can operate safely and effectively by guaranteeing that staff members have the appropriate training that is routinely evaluated and updated.

Every aspect of working at the facility should be covered in training, including handling and storing items, using the various tools and equipment correctly, maintaining good personal hygiene, facility sanitation needs, and much more. Employees in a pet food processing facility are equipped to manage everything required to maintain food safety with the help of proper training.

Store Ingredients Properly

In order to avoid the formation of bacteria, different substances must be stored using different techniques.

Everything should have a place to be stored, preferably in containers that can be sealed tightly. Products that are not kept in tightly sealed containers risk spoiling or luring insects and rodents that transmit disease-causing microorganisms.

Additionally, ingredients require accurate labelling so that workers can correctly identify and rotate product, minimising errors and ensuring that good first in, first out (FIFO) protocols are followed. To keep track of the shelf life, labels should specify the nature of a component or product as well as its production date.If such precautions are required, good labelling practises also assist investigators in tracing the source of contamination.

Set up Appropriate Floor Drainage

In order to keep a facility dry, clean, and free of bacteria and pollution, floor drainage is crucial. For instance, a facility's drainage system is the cause of 70% of positive listeria screenings, demonstrating how crucial it is to pick the right kind of drains.

FoodSafe Drains is the best choice for pet food production facilities because of their pre-sloped, linear, and grate-free drainage systems. Our drains are incredibly durable because they are constructed of stainless steel. Slot drains from FoodSafe Drains are resistant to temperature, corrosion, and germs because to the stainless steel construction of items like the 10,000 Series.

Additionally, there are no 90-degree angles in these drains, preventing any bacterial harbour spots.

Ensure that the space is Clean

Every facility's top goal should be cleanliness, in addition to providing excellent products. Each day, workers are expected to properly clean the building, including the floors and lights. They should make sure that none of the surfaces contain food particles or leftover microorganisms that can encourage the growth of bacteria.

Cleaning of the building goes beyond only the areas you can see and use every day. To make sure that no leftover trash is left in the channel, where it might draw bugs and support the growth of mould or other sorts of contamination, the drainage system also needs to be thoroughly cleaned.

To keep a system sufficiently sanitised, even systems like Slot Drain that are resistant to bacteria require daily cleaning. Cleaning the drain channel is quick and straightforward thanks to the brush and paddle tools, and FoodSafe Slot Drains have clean-in-place features like our Flush-Flo attachment, which permits a waterline connection for quick flushing of the channel.

Apply Best Practices For Layout

The plan should start with the raw materials and end with the finished product, just like in any other facility that produces food. The spread of bacteria and contamination to other areas of the facility is minimised by adhering to this protocol, thus doing otherwise is crucial. The appropriate structure also reduces the likelihood of production errors and makes the workplace safer for the personnel.

Furthermore, Pets have always been our friends, but they have evolved into much more. A pet should receive the utmost care because it is a member of the family. Without safe food, a pet may experience a wide range of health problems. In rare situations, problems with pet food safety may even result in permanent health problems and death.

Facilities can provide the best safety and sanitation possible by enhancing current procedures and putting in place additional safety measures. The facility, its staff, and—most importantly—the animals that are consuming the food will all be safeguarded by the appropriate procedures.

Companies ensure safety of Pet Food

Pet food producers are aware that food safety is essential to delivering wholesome food that supports good ageing in pets and fosters consumer confidence.

Government and industry laws that govern the production of pet food, including those relating to ingredients, plant hygiene, and product storage, must be followed by businesses.

Reputable businesses implement a hazard management programme that finds, assesses, mitigates, and keeps an eye on potential risks to the safety of their products. The programme is applicable to every step of the production process, from choosing the raw materials through producing the finished good.

To ensure that quality and safety standards are fulfilled, pet food producers employ a system of safety and quality checks, beginning with supplier audits, ingredient deliveries, and continuing all the way through production until the product leaves the plant.

Some pet food manufacturers offer important retailers education and training on proper food handling and storage techniques that help guarantee the quality of pet food.

Chapter 9

Trends Shaping Pet Nutrition: Hype vs. Health

A growing understanding of the significance of pets' health and wellbeing has led to a remarkable revolution in the pet feeding industry in recent years. Demand for premium pet food and nutrition has increased as more people view their furry friends as essential family members. However, a division between trends that promise game-changing advantages and those that really prioritise the health of our cherished pets has formed within this quickly expanding landscape. This conflict between marketing hype and human health has produced questions and disagreements about the ideal method of pet nutrition.

Now we will discuss some important points about it. These are;

- Holistic Wellness
- The Protein Predicament
- Personalization through Technology
- The Grain-Free Conundrum
- The Role of Supplements

Holistic Wellness

The term "holistic care" refers to the management of a pet as a whole, taking into account its diet, environment, genetics, behaviour, and medical history. Love, empathy, respect, and seeing an animal as an individual are at the core of holistic thinking.

Holistic means considering each aspect of a dog's health.

We take a "holistic" approach to medicine by taking into account each dog's overall health, way of life, and diet in order to identify their specific problem or problems and develop a health programme that will improve their quality of life.

The Protein Predicament

Putting more emphasis on high-protein foods for pets is another idea that has gained traction. Many pet feeds now feature increased protein content due to the belief that animals thrive on diets high in protein that are similar to their ancestors' diets. Although excessive amounts of protein may cause health problems, such as kidney strain in cats and dogs, they are still necessary for pets. This emphasises the necessity for a balanced strategy and customised feeding schedules that take breed, age, and activity level into account.

Personalization through Technology

Technology developments have resulted in a new era of individualised pet nutrition. Businesses provide services to provide custom meals for pets based on genetic analysis. Although this innovation shows promise, concerns about the accuracy of these assessments and how much nutritional requirements are really determined by genetics persist. Responsible pet owners must discern between unsupported claims and science-based personalisation.

The Grain-Free Conundrum

Many grain-free dog and cat meals are marketed to customers as being healthier than feeding grains. This is untrue and some dogs and cats may become unwell as a result. Giving dogs or cats a diet devoid of grains has no physiological or medicinal justification.

There may be a medical need to restrict the source of carbohydrates in a dog or cat's diet if they have a specific food allergy. For certain animals, this can be accomplished by feeding them a grain-free diet. An anti-corn sentiment gave rise to the grain-free craze. Corn was taken out of the dog food as a source of carbohydrates since it was thought that some dogs with food allergies would react to it. Tubers (potatoes and sweet potatoes) and legumes (peas and lentils) were used as the new source of carbohydrates; these meals were designated as "grain-free." The idea that maize is bad has no basis in reality and is a fallacy. Pet food may contain grains such as corn, soy, wheat, rice, barley, or other grains.

While some dogs or cats may develop food allergies to these sources, most animals have no trouble handling grains. Since grass is a grain, many cats and dogs will eat it. Peas, lentils, other legume seeds, or potatoes will serve as the main sources of carbohydrates in the grain-free dishes.

The Role of Supplements

As with humans, the purpose of pet supplements for animals is to supplement a diet deficient in nutrients in order to meet animal demands, typically for maintenance, development, pregnancy, or lactation. Supplements can provide extra vitamins that an animal's diet might be lacking.

At last, The most important thing you can do for your pet is to take care of them, even though there are many other methods to show them that you care. Maintain your schedule and make sure your pet receives food that is nutrient-rich. To keep your pet interested, take them on a walk or buy them an enjoyable new gift.